The Low Glucose Load, Low Blood Sugar Diet

John Rope

Simple Information Publishing

John Rope is a clinical psychologist who has worked in the British National Health Service and in private practice in Spain.

His interest in weight control began when he was diagnosed with angina and told he had to keep his weight down. When he found the diet provided by the hospital caused him to put on weight, he decided to look at the science. The results of that research are in this book.

He is now symptom free and living a healthy happy and slim life in Wiltshire UK .

The Low Glucose Load, Low Blood Sugar Diet

A guide to the losing weight easily

John Rope

A diet which is flexible

A diet which can fit into your life

A gentle way of weight control

Simple Information Publishing

Thank you for reading this book. It is part of the Simple Nutrition Series covering various aspects of nutrition and weight control. They are designed on a modular basis so that key elements are included with each topic, at least in brief form, to keep the length of the book down and prevent the user having to refer to another book for explanation all the time. Obviously a book in the series covering that topic will be more informative and detailed.

Other Books in the Simple Nutrition Series by John Rope Your Future Fat or Slim? (No longer in print)

Sugar Free-Dom How To Kick The Sugar Demon Out Of Your Life *

Why Diets Don't Work (And What We Can Do About It)*

Be Your Own Diet Expert*

The Psychology Of Weight Loss*

How To Start Intermittent Fasting A Simple Guide (Available soon)

Starting A Low Carb Diet A Beginners Guide (Available soon)

The Great Diet Conspiracy (Available soon)

Design Your Own Diet (Available soon)*
* Work Book/Journal available

Published by Simple Information Publishing

Foreword

The common prejudice about overweight people, they are fat, lazy and eat too much, received a massive knockout blow when Gary Taubes published his seminal book, 'Good Calories, Bad Calories' in 2007 (published as 'The Diet Delusion' in the UK) . To quote him:-

"People who are overweight are assumed to overeat and are labelled as greedy, whereas in terms of calories, many eat less than the generally recommended level of 2000-2400 calories per day and remain overweight. Thin people who eat far more than 2400 calories (*and stay slim-my addition)* are labelled as 'hearty eaters' but should be grossly overweight according to the traditional theory."

This book is my attempt to do something, no matter how small, about the unfairness our society meets out to overweight people. If it helps to redress some of the wrong done to so many weight sufferers over the years, then I am happy.

To my darling wife Barbara

Table Of Contents

Introduction

In 2013 designed own diet which I published in 2014. I wanted a method of understanding and eating food which would help me to lose weight but be flexible and easy to keep to. This diet gave me what I needed. I have never had a problem putting on weight, I just ate carbs and sugar! As a result I was able to test various diet regimes because if a diet didn't work I could get back to my 'working weight' in reasonable time using my diet.

This diet is considerably simpler than my previous diet, easier to understand and follow. Keeping the 'glucose load* of your food to a minimum allows the natural energy regulation of the body to take over, so you use ingested food as fuel and then give your body time to burn stored fat as energy. It also gives your endocrine system a holiday and allows you to recover from diseases like insulin resistance.**

Hunger is not a problem on the diet because you can eat a nutritious and satisfying diet and still lose weight.

* Explained below. ** The cause of overweight. For more details than there is space for here see my book 'Be your own diet expert' available on Kindle.

Chapter 1

Why Control Blood Glucose?

Blood glucose and insulin

We must control blood glucose because blood glucose begets the hormone insulin. Insulin is the hormone which governs fat accumulation and we must control that if we wish to lose weight.

Insulin packs the glucose energy in the blood stream into the cells of the body, Foods which contain lots of carbs, convertible into blood glucose, give rise to blood glucose spikes which stimulate the pancreas to release an equivalent about of insulin leading to insulin spikes.

Once the level of blood glucose has been reduced sufficiently there is often a residual amount of insulin in the blood. If the process is repeated too often the normal levels of insulin in the blood rise to such an extent no fat can be burned. In fact excess glucose is stored as fat. Insulin is the fat storage hormone.

All carbohydrates except fibre are converted into blood glucose. Some low carb diets focus on the total carb content which is measured by something called the glucose index or Gi. All foods are compared with an equal amount of glucose which has a GL of 100.

Because of fibre and the structure of some foods only some of the carb content is actually available for glucose production. This is measured by glucose load or GL which is calculated from the Gi.

In a nutshell: Insulin is he fat storage hormone and is released in response to rises in blood glucose. The glucose load or GL of a food is a measure of the amount of blood glucose produced by eating the carbohydrate contained in a serving of the food.

Insulin Resistance

Insulin resistance refers to the inability of cells to accept more glucose with normal blood levels of insulin, despite large amounts of glucose remaining in the blood stream. This causes the pancreas, which makes insulin, to produce more and more insulin to force energy into the cells which eventually become totally resistant to the its effects.

With the normal cells blocked there is no other place for the glucose to go other than the fat cells which remain open 24/7.

If this goes on the pancreas becomes unable to produce insulin in sufficient amounts to counteract the blood glucose, even in normal quantities, and blood glucose levels rise dramatically.

We have become diabetic.

Examples

Foods with a high glucose load (GL) of greater than 20

Macn'cheese 52

Dried dates 43

Pancake 39

Foods with a low glucose load (GL) of less than 11

Ice cream 8

Green peas boiled 3

Tomatoes raw 1

Some foods which have a high glucose index but a low glucose load. This means foods which simple low glucose index diets would forbid are allowed in moderation on a low GL diet. This makes a low GL diet much more flexible than a straight carb reduction diet based on glucose index.

Example	Gi	GL	
Carrots	47	3	
Garden peas	48	3	
Oranges	42	5	

What these low glucose load foods do is to release their carbs slowly so the glucose energy they contain reaches the blood stream over a longer period of time. This means less insulin is produced and it diminishes more quickly, leaving the way clear for fat burning.

In a nutshell: It is the glycemic load, or GL, of a food which controls insulin production and therefore fat accumulation. It is the time over which glucose is released to the blood stream, which is critical to controlling our insulin response to carbohydrates.

Adding up the GL of foods

Meals on the other hand are a jungle of high and low GL foods for the unaware. In order to navigate our way through the jungle of we to first of all become adept at recognising the high and low components of any meal and adjusting content and portion sizes to suit us.

Just as some foods will be off our list, even in small portions, so some meals particular foods will be off because of the cumulative effect of GL values in the meal. This does not mean you cannot eat that food next day or next week. If it doesn't take you over your limit on a particular day then it can be eaten. Try to spread your GL allowance over the day to keep insulin levels down

This means we will need to start by calculating the GL value of the most common or typical meals we eat at home by adding together the GL's of all the components and adjusting them to keep within a set limit of GL units.

A small amount of food with a high GL in a meal will quickly produce a high blood glucose spike and a great deal of insulin, effectively blocking the body's fat burning and turning excess fuel into fat for a time. We need to dilute the effects of these high GL foods by replacing them with low GL ones.

You will be given a maximum total for your day's GL intake of 40 and you will need to keep track of the GL's of food you eat in a small notebook you can carry around in your pocket or purse (handbag).

Example

Roast beef, Carrots, potatoes and peas

GLs:- Roast beef 0, carrots 2, potatoes 26, peas 3.

Total 31. Nearly all your daily allowance in one meal.

Whereas:

Roast beef 0, carrots 2, cabbage 0. Cauliflower 0

Total 2

A filling meal, leaving plenty of room for other courses or meals.

Another advantage of the diet is leaving it for any reason. You do not have to feel guilty about an occasional foray into unhealthy eating; just return to the diet and reduce your GL allowance for a few days.

Hunger
It is unlikely you will experience hunger on the diet after the first two days, except for a half hour just before usual mealtimes, as your body learns to switch from glucose power to fat burning power. Once you have started to regain normal metabolic functioning even that will disappear. No need to feel guilty.

The range of foods you can eat on al low GL diet is much greater than on low carb or low fat diets. It must still be considered a low carb diet but it has much more flexibility for eating with the family, eating out and attending celebrations.

As you regulate your carbohydrate intake and your resting insulin levels drop, your body will manage the transition from fat creation/deposition to fat burning smoothly because that is how our bodies are designed.

Keeping your insulin levels low and avoiding sugar and processed carbs are the keys to weight control, avoiding the gnawing hunger associated with low calorie diets.

By allowing a broader spectrum of low GL food any residual hunger rapidly disappears on the diet.

In a nutshell: By keeping the glucose load of our meals low we allow glucose to be dealt with effectively by our body, preventing high insulin responses. By learning to recognise low and high GL foods we can develop our own safe choices and avoid harmful ones without feeling hungry.

Eating out

You are allowed an extra allowance for eating out. You can lower GL of the food you eat the day after eat outing and then go back to your usual GL limit the following day without any detriment to the program. Provided you at least stick to the simple rules of the diet most of the time, you should be O.K. for the occasional, controlled celebration.

Having said that, the fact the diet is designed not to disrupt your lifestyle in the way some 'diets' do, still means some changes are to be made. The gentle nature of the program allows for steady lifestyle adjustments, to a more healthy way of eating. The basic rule still applies- If you keep doing what you have been doing, you will keep getting what you have been getting-FAT!

My message is change can be easy, change can be fun and change can keep you alive.

In a nutshell: Eating out can be coped with by reducing your GL limit the day after the non diet day. You will need some lifestyle changes but once you get going it is going to be fun!

About You

Have you tried to diet many times in the past and either given up or put the weight you lost back on shortly after ending the diet?

Have you ever been diagnosed with obesity, pre-diabetes, diabetes heart disease, stroke or polycystic ovarian syndrome?

Is you waist measurement bigger than your hips?

Do you have cravings for sugary things and foods with a high sugar content like cakes, biscuits or 'savouries' such as pizzas, fish and chips or burgers?

If you have answered yes to any one of these questions you may have insulin resistance. If you are insulin resistant you will have difficulty loosing weight and the insulin resistance will be the reason you may have illnesses such as those above.

Chapter 2

Setting Sensible Goals and Targets

What is a sensible goal?

Setting sensible goals and targets and patience are essential to successful weight loss.

Don't set your overall goal weight to achieve an unachievable shape! If you are 40+ it is unlikely you will achieve the figure you had when you were 20, whether you are male or female.

Your targets for weight loss should be set in accordance with your body shape and fitness level. My shape is average height but a bit chunky and so even at my ideal weight I am not going to look tall, slim and elegant; it is a pity but there you are! Equally there is no point setting an average weight if you want to be into sport or personal fitness to a degree which increases your muscle mass above average and raises your weight because of the higher density of muscle to that of fat.

For the same reason you may not lose weight at all for a time or even gain weight because you have put on muscle mass at the same time as you lose fat. Check your waist size to see if this is true. If your waist size is the same or less you have lost fat.

The rate at which you lose weight will depend on your starting weight, the heavier you are the more you will loose at first but this slows down. Don't expect to loose more than 2 to 3 pounds a week* at first and expect that to slow down as you lose weight. The plus side is you won't be hungry either.

These are realistic levels of true weight loss. Any more and you can say goodbye to muscle as well as fat. By setting your expectations at this level you are going to be avoiding disappointment and you will prepare yourself for the long haul which is sustainable and permanent weight loss.

After all you didn't put the weight on in two weeks did you?

*An exception to this rule is the first two or three weeks when higher weight loss may be achieved. This is due to the loss of water weight bound up with glucose stored as a starch called glycogen contained in the liver and muscles. Similarly if you go back to eating a lot high GL carbs your weight will rise as excess glucose is converted into starch.

In a nutshell: Trimming your expectations of expected weight loss to realistic levels is important to avoid disappointment. Set your sights from the beginning on a long haul. What took maybe twenty years to achieve will not disappear over night.

Chapter 3

Starting The diet

Although all carbohydrates absorbed by the digestive system generate glucose in the blood, not all of the carbohydrate we eat is able to be absorbed, since it is in the form of fibre which is not absorbed by the small intestine and performs other important functions. Foods with more fibre are our friends along with other low GL foods.

The diet works by allowing the body's natural weight control mechanisms to take over while avoiding the disruption to life style caused by crash diets, and the flip flop back to previous bad eating habits when you crash out again.

One of the most difficult parts of losing weight, in the traditional way, is the need to maintain a different feeding regime from the rest of the family. Another is the experience of such things as hunger, weakness and lethargy at times, often getting worse, not better, as time goes on. This can lead to an eating rebound at the end of the weight reduction program, whereby people overindulge in all of the forbidden foods of the past weeks and rapidly regain the weight they lost. The low GL diet avoids this by being a whole life diet plan, allowing healthy levels of calorie intake and

About You

You will find on line many weight calculators which take into account your height, sexing age. Although not the be all and end all of dieting, such measures make a sensible start for an overall goal.

As a general guide the following are average weights for both men and women.

Men and Women

Height	Av weight Lbs
5ft	107-112
5ft 1 inch	111-116
5ft 2 inch	115-120
5ft 3 inch	120-126
5ft 4 inch	122-128
5ft 5 inch	126-132
5ft 6 inch	130-136
5ft 7inch	134-140
5ft 8 inch	138-144
5ft 9 inch	142-149
5ft 10 inch	146-153
6 ft	154-162
6ft 1 inch	159-166
6ft 2 inch	163-171

These are averages and if you consult an ideal weight chart it will vary these according to your body build age and sex.

satiety, fitting easily into a modern lifestyle. Add to that the elimination of 'failure' and you have the perfect solution to overweight and the metabolic syndrome.

At no time should you feel hungry, or bloated or constipated. You can vary the GL of your food and depending on your plans. So you could move from the very low GL on a day before and event, say a dinner date, to high gL the ay after. In this way you can eat more normally in the evening and still maintain your momentum of weight loss.

You are allowed an extra allowance of 5 GL for eating out. You can mix and match your days without any detriment to the program. Provided you at least stick to the simple rules of the inside lane 90% of the time, you should be O.K. for the occasional, controlled celebration.

Having said that, the fact the diet is designed not to disrupt your lifestyle in the way some 'diets' do, still means some changes are to be made. The idea is the gentle nature of the program allows for steady lifestyle adjustments, to a more healthy way of eating. The basic rule still applies- If you keep doing what you have been doing, you will keep getting what you have been getting-FAT!

We are designed to burn most of our day's production of body fat at night while we are sleeping. If we are overweight this is probably not the case. By limiting the amount of glucose in our blood steam, the diet extends the nocturnal fat burning time by two to three times normal.

In the initial weight reduction phase the only carbs which are eaten are low GL carbs. Once a significant amount of weight (30% of target weight) has been lost, naughty carbs such as potatoes, rice and bread can be eaten in reduced amounts.

I must emphasise any manufactured food or beverage should be treated as out of bounds for the purposes of staying on the weight reduction phase of the program.

During the initial weight reduction phase, zero manufactured food is the only safe number. If you must have a particular manufactured food, then investigate it closely and try to calculate its GL before you eat any of it. If you cannot do this, then you have temporarily come off the diet.

In a nutshell: To make use of the body's nocturnal fat burning we need to keep our glucose levels low, only eating low GL foods. This means zero manufactured food.

The low glucose load diet an easy start guide

Plan it first, don't jump straight in:-

Look at the food lists and decide which items you want to eliminate from your cupboards and which you need to stock up on.

This can be difficult if you are the only person who is on a this diet in the family. However it can can fit around a more 'normal 'diet 'so think about the meals you prepare and add low GL to them. You eat the low GL and others eat the rest.

For example if you normally prepare potatoes or rice for a meal prepare some cauliflower or cauliflower rice as well. You eat the cauliflower and ignore the potatoes or rice and everyone else eats the potatoes and is free to have cauliflower if the want.

Go through the foods you will be eating and find out the GL of a normal portion using the tables below.

Plan your start time: Whatever you do don't start a diet just after the holidays when you are annoyed or even feeling angry with yourself for putting on weight again. The first of January is no better than any other day and worse than most to redesign your whole life diet.

Decide how much weight you need to lose and calculate 30% of that amount so you know when you can start

including special cases like French fries or rice into your diet.

Try it out on a few typical meals before you announce you are on a diet. Sort out any problems before your nearest and dearest are expecting results.

Select a start date to suite you.

When you have done your planning and given the meals a dry run then the only thing left is to find a convenient time to suit you. Avoid, as far as possible, holidays, visitors and celebrations in the first two weeks. Once you have bedded into the diet you will be able to take account of them. The winter holiday celebrations can stretch over several weeks and it is a good idea to try to launch the new you before they start. In the case of the USA before Thanksgiving.

Expect your progress to be slow, because if you lose weight fast you are in danger of telling your body you are in a starvation situation and triggering defence mechanisms which slow down your metabolism and put a stop to weight loss. Remember, the first few pounds will be water loss.

Avoid all sugars and commercially produced foods and drinks. Drink water, tea and coffee. Eat as much as you like of high fibre leafy vegetables with low GL like greens, cauliflower, broccoli and carrots.

Drink lots of fluids- try to drink 6 extra glasses (2 litres) of water a day to flush the system. Our bodies are homeostatic mechanisms. Which means they adjust to changes and try to bring the body back to a normal state.

When you are losing weight your will be generating lots of by-products and releasing poisons stored in your fat. These need to be eliminated from the body in the normal way via the kidneys. If you do not flush the kidneys enough then the body will retain water to keep the body concentrations of these waste products to a minimum. Hence, perversely, we may put on weight because of this homeostatic mechanism.

In a nutshell: Design your entry into the diet carefully and prepare yourself for a long haul. Too many diets fail because they don't mentally prepare people for the road ahead. Take care of housekeeping like drinking plenty of water. Be prepared!

About You

Do some homework based on the previous chapter and make a note below:

A. Current weight.

B. Target weight

C. Total to lose lbs or kilos

D. 30% of total

Weight at which I can start using
special cases (A-D)

=

Expected time (months) to
Target weight = C(lbs)/4*

=

*You will lose more quickly at first but this will slow down as you progress. 4Lbs is a good estimate of an average per month.

Chapter 4

The Low Glucose Load Diet

Rules

1. Eat a total GL of 40 or less a day. To begin with (until you have lost 30% of your target weight) you are strongly advised to avoid processed foods and any white vegetables from the high GL list. Eat your vegetables from the list of foods with a GL of 5 or less. You can eat as many portions of these as your daily allowance permits but try to spread you eating over the day.

2. Vegetables and fruit with a GL of less than 3 are zero rated, and can be eaten freely.

3. You may eat protein at any mealtime in the day up to a maximum of 130 grams a day; any meat, fish, Quorn, TVP, tofu, eggs, cheese, **but not legumes (beans etc.).** Nuts need to be limited to one or two handfuls and are best used as a snack or to assuage hunger.

4. It is best to cut out alcohol entirely until you have started to lose a significant amount of weight, say 30% of the weight you wish to lose. If you want to lose 3 stones for instance, then wait until you have lost 1 stone before reintroducing alcohol. Even then, keep it to an occasional treat, say one

small glass of wine or beer one to two times a week up to a maximum four glasses per week.

5. Breakfast can be either low carb or omitted (fasted).

If you follow these rules then you should start to lose some weight each week, but this is a gentle weight loss program and so don't expect too much.

Examples

For extra clarity, I have worked through some examples of typical meals before and after entering the diet below.

Breakfast

Before entering the diet.

Example 1: Orange juice (concentrated*) followed by Cornflakes followed by two slices of toast and marmalade. Total GL=21+17+11= 49.

*Concentrated fruit juice is a double problem in that it may contain added sugar.

Example 2: Black coffee, with 2 eggs bacon and 2 sausages, with two slices of toast.

Total GL =17 (for the toast).

Note: I have ignored the possible GL contribution of the sausages since this has to be calculated for each individual brand, depending on the carb content and the calculated GL of that content.

After entering the diet

Example 1: Half grapefruit followed by 2 boiled eggs and coffee.

Total GL= 0+0+0= 0 (grapefruit and coffee are zero rated)

Example 2: Coffee with 2 eggs, bacon

Total GL= 0+0= 0.
Lunch

Before entering the diet

Example 3: A rye bread sandwich with, ham and mayonnaise, followed by a piece of plain sponge cake. Total GL = 14+18=32 (for the bread and cake).

Example 4: Office canteen meal; Roast pork with roast potatoes peas and apple sauce, followed by pineapple upside down cake and a generous helping of custard (made from powder not fresh eggs). Total GL = 20+15+5=40.

After entering the diet

Example 3: Ham salad with a little mayonnaise, followed by a dessert of natural yoghurt and fresh blueberries. Total GL =0.

Example 4: Office canteen meal; Roast pork with carrots and peas followed by strawberries and (unsweetened) cream. Total GL =3.

And so on.

Switching to low GL can make a big difference in carbohydrate intake while keeping a good range of foods available.

The diet allows you to go on eating many of the things you like by eating them in moderation (having regard to the glucose load). You can theoretically still lose weight on a near normal calorie intake but one based on low GL foods. However a calorie reduction of 20% to 25% is advisable. In this respect a phone app like 'Lose it'or' 'My Fitness Pal' may be very helpful.

At first you may feel the need to snack between meals and you can do this on low carb foods with a GL of 3 or less, from the snack list below. You can do this twice per day between meals. If you snack more than twice you must add all those extra instances to the GL of the next meal. Try to phase out snacks as early as possible.

In a nutshell: You must monitor your GL intake to keep below 40GL. Snacks are allowed but only from the snack list. Try to phase these out.

Chapter 5

Snacks and Special Cases

Snacks

One secret of dieting is not to snack and you should try to eliminate these entirely. Better to add these to your actual meals. But if you need something a little extra at first you can eat one of the following twice a day:-

One Quorn sausage or burger, eaten without accompaniments or sauces. I have calculated the maximum GL of one sausage or burger to be 2.5. If you eat more than one, you must add their combined GL to the GL of the next meal.

Note: this applies only to the original Quorn sausages, not to any newer versions which contain too much sugar and should be avoided at all costs.

One whole meat sausage or burger, guaranteed to be made from around ninety percent ground meat and seasoning, and with no more than two percent bread or other carbohydrates as fillers, without accompaniment or sauces.

Again, if you have more than one, their combined GL must be added to the GL of the next meal. See your butcher or the information on the packet. Beware added sugars in packet sausages.

One or two teaspoonful's of nut butter-not peanut butter.

A small apple, pear, orange or a portion of acid fruits (berries, citrus, plums etc).

A small bag or handful of nuts (not cashews or peanuts).

Cheese 100 grams (no bread).
A medium sized carrot or bell pepper eaten with some guacamole or hummus dip.

A bowl of strawberries or cherries (or any other berry fruit) and cream.

One or two dessert spoonfuls of butter or coconut oil can assuage hunger, encourage fat burning and keep your insulin levels down. This is a good replacement breakfast.

Special cases-some examples
For after you have lost 30% of your target loss

A small baked potato.

Normal GL of 150 gram portion size is 26.

GL of 26 grams= 5.

This is about the size of a small computer mouse. Check it on your scales!

About You

Check your understanding of the terms of the low GL diet.

Glucose load is?

1. The amount of glucose in a meal.

2. The amount of sugar you put in your tea or coffee.

3. The amount of glucose released into the blood by a standard amount of a food compared with the same quantity of glucose.

Your glucose limit is?

1. The GL of each meal.

2. The limit to the total GL of all meals eaten in one day.

3. The total of the GL's of all meals eaten in a week.

Glucose load is?

!. The same as glucose index.

2. More relevant than glucose index.

3. Less accurate than glucose index.

Correct answers 3,2,2.

Rice, white, brown and wild

Normal GL of 150 gram portion is 26.

GL 5= 26 grams (wet weight)

This is a small portion but better than none, if you like white rice. Surprisingly brown rice and wild rice are exactly the same and must similarly be decreased to 26 gram portion sizes. An alternative to rice is cauliflower rice made by grating the cauliflower and cooking in the microwave. It takes longer to prepare but cooks in less than five minutes.

French-fries or chips(UK).

Normal GL of 150 gram portion= 22.

GL of 31 grams= 5 GL.

Because this is a fat/carb combination the actual recommendation is 16 grams.

This is one tenth of a normal portion, about a very small handful. I would encourage you not to eat french-fries except on very rare occasions.

In all cases, do not go by your idea of a normal portion. Measure it out and make sure. In a short time your eye will tell you how much to eat.

Get used to leaving some carbs on your plate. If your plate is clean you won't get lean.

Try to keep these special cases to once or twice a week perhaps to reward yourself for something, like staying in the GL guidelines when out at a restaurant.

If you stop losing weight, or start to put on weight when you begin to allow special cases then avoid all white carbs until you have achieved all of your desired weight loss and then only if you do not start to put on weight again.

In a nutshell: Special cases are just that, they are occasional treats When you are with the over caring aunt who insists you have some potato, accept her offer and leave the portion you are not allowed. Make sure you ask for more cauliflower or broccoli, to reassure her you are eating well.

Eating in restaurants

If you are eating out, the maximum GL allowed for a the day is increased to 45. You are advised to do this only once a week.

If you eat out more frequently, the meal limit for all other occasions remains whatever will keep you within the daily limit of GL 40.

Anything more than these allowances and you have temporarily left the diet and you need to reduce your GL allowance next day and perhaps for one or two days.

I have found restaurants will swop out French fries or sautéd potatoes for green vegetables or salad. The English staple of fish and chips can be coped with by asking if they will cook the fish on a grill without batter. This is sometimes the gluten free option on a menu. Alternatively ask for a separate plate to put the batter on leaving steamed fish.

In a nutshell: Eating out requires ingenuity and some boldness to ask for things not on the menu but most restaurants are happy to help.

If you do not lose much weight at first

If you have not lost much weight at the end of four weeks, less than six pounds, you may be someone who has a higher than normal insulin response or 'insulin resistance', leading to prolonged blocking of the fat burning process. You will need to do the following:-

First, check the portion sizes of all the carbs you have been eating and make sure you have them correct. If they were too high then try the correct portion sizes for couple of weeks and re-weigh yourself. You should not

be eating anything containing on the high cabs list until you have lost 30% of your target weight loss.

Second, if you are still not losing weight and your portion sizes were correct, review your eating between meals. Are all of your snacks from the recommended list above? If not, cut out anything you have been eating which is not on the list. Just one sugary candy or biscuit between breakfast and lunch could interfere with the whole of that day's fat burning process.

Third, reduce your daily GL limit by 30% for a week. If you still don't lose weight, you may need to use consider moving towards a full blown ketogenic diet. If you consider this then my book 'How To Begin a Ketogenic Diet A Simple Guide' will be available soon on Kindle

Don't forget to drink plenty of water. Over the day you should try to consume six glasses of water as well as your normal coffee and tea.

In a nutshell: If this diet isn't working for you you may need a Ketogenic diet. If so consider this as training.

Chapter 6

Temporarily Leaving the diet

Once you have become familiar with the regime of the diet, and the portion sizes of permitted carbs, you will find most special occasions, such as parties and restaurant meals can be coped with within the parameters of the diet.

On these occasions, the special cases of the diet can come in handy. High GL foods like French-fries, pasta, batter and rice can be eaten, in reduced portions, without leaving the diet. The danger here is, the total GL for the meal will take you above the permitted restaurant upper limit of 45 GL because of the preponderance of high GL foods and the number of courses. In that case you have temporarily left the diet.

As you become used to the diet you will find it easy to omit certain foods or courses because your addictive drive to eat food will have gone.

If you leave diet don't panic, after all if you left the freeway/motorway to stop at services, you would not panic about your journey. You would rejoin the motorway and put on a bit of speed to make up for the lost time in the services.

That is exactly what you do when you leave the diet, you just move to a lower G limit for a few days to regain some speed.

In a nutshell: The diet is rather like hotel California, you can check out any time you like but you need never leave. This flexibility means there is no such thing as failure on the diet. Just different speeds.

Example of leaving the diet
Extreme case, lunch out.

Main meal, Lasagne.

Constituents		Weight gms	GL
Large Portion of pasta		200	30
French fries		200	34
Other constituents		Estimate	30
Total estimated GL			94

Result, you have left the diet.

The carbs you have eaten will be stored as glycogen in your liver and you will need to burn them off before you can resume fat burning.

In this case the carb intake is very high and so it would be advisable to avoid carbs as much as possible for a couple of days. Some light fasting would also get things back on track. See my book

About The Diet

I discovered a long time ago I wasn't perfect and I do not expect you to be so either.

Don't worry if things go awry one day, you can recover very easily next day. The human weight control system is so complex and sophisticated you could even find you have lost weight the day after a difficult day.

What matters is continuing adjustment of your lifestyle and your eating habits towards a better, healthier way of eating and living.

Studies of various diets show people do not keep to the strict bounds of a diet from the beginning. This is why I have designed this diet to be very flexible. Of course you can't keep to the letter of the diet, day in and day out but if you try and keep as close to it as possible, it will work for you.

available soon on Kindle.

If you are unsure about the portions and constituents of a meal, assume you have left the diet anyway and resume with a lower GL limit the day after the meal. I would recommend a GL limit if 20.

You could, of course, make this your only meal of the day, effectively fasting before and after to compensate. If you skip breakfast on the day you extend your overnight fast, and if you skip dinner you commence your next overnight fat burning sooner. +

In a nutshell: If you cannot avoid eating high GL food just compensate for it by moving to a lower GL limit next day.

Cheat Days

Carb days, or 'cheat days' as they are sometimes called, mean eating a lot of carbs on one or two days a week to boost your metabolic rate. A Cornell University study claims it is the rhythm of weight gain and loss which is important. For most people weight gain at weekends is normal and should not be seen as a reversal of a diet.

Their subjects were men and women with poorly regulated endocrine systems and so their study at least passed the test of dealing with the most difficult cases.

They conclude that weekdays are when you lose weight and some degree of 'splurging' which can happen at weekends is no bad thing.

This has been interpreted by some to mean eating carbs ad. lib. at weekends, can boost your metabolism to achieve greater weight loss than you would slavishly sticking to a diet.

Even moderate calorie reduction such as we have observed in the best diets can lead to a suppression of metabolic rate and this can persist for a long time after the diet is terminated. The occasional boost to metabolism, from forays into the forbidden carbs, may indeed be beneficial. More research is needed.

There is already a model for this phenomenon in some of the intermittent fasting regimes. In these people typically eat normally for say three or four days a week and then fast on 600 to 800 calories for the remainder and these are spread throughout the week.

The fast days are the 'diet' part of the regime and the non fasting days are the 'cheat' days.

This method produces impressive results but there is no control over how many calories are omitted on diet days. Dr Krista Varady who has researched this over a number of years holds that 25% of normal calories is necessary to get results and it is just possible other regimes benefit from this on/off approach.

The idea coming off your diet once a week actually helps rather than hinders your weight loss will be a comfort to many. However, not everybody follows this weekly pattern and you could try it if your weight is normally lower on a Friday evening than on Sunday evening. If it stays the same or goes up you may be an individual who would put on weight with this trick.

Other regimes claimed to work in a similar manner include skipping breakfast everyday and fasting until say 12 p.m. and then only eating in an 8 hour window until 8 p.m., giving a 16/8 hour fast/ eat cycle. I frequently employ this method although I prefer to restrict eating to a window between 1 p.m. and 6 p.m. which it helps keep my weight in check while allowing me freedom to eat more liberally at weekends.

In a nutshell: Alternating or occasional deliberate forays into higher carb eating may suit some people but it is best to understand the basis of theses approaches.

Chapter 7

Maintenance

Once you have achieved the results you want from weight loss it is time to think about maintenance.

Maintenance is not a matter of leaving the diet altogether but rather of expanding your carb intake sensibly in a way which suites you. It is still necessary to control the intake of processed carbs. Somewhere between 55 and 65 total GL per day is a good area but you will have to explore this for yourself.

You could continue to expand your carbs slowly and allow yourself just an occasional high GL day (though not excessive).

This makes eating out easier and if you think you have gone a bit too far, you can eat low GL the next day.

You may find this method does not suit you, and that you are better keeping carbs fairly low all day by keeping all GLs, say, to 15 per meal, with two 5GI Snacks with a total for the day of 55. The diet is very flexible. What you must not do, is to come off the diet altogether. Remember this is not a diet; this is a permanent weight control system and a safe way to live.

If you find your weight creeping up go back to a

Using A Weight Loss App

You may find it useful to use an app such as My Fitness Pal or Lose It. They do not, unfortunately, give you GL measures but they do give you total carbs, fibre and available carbs.

Obviously not al carbs are the same but if you use the available carbs figure for a meal in grams and multiply that by .70%which is a rough GL of things like rice, potatoes and sugar it will give you an estimate of the total GL impact of the meal.

As in the example below:

Total carbs=90 grams

Fibre =50 grams

Available carbs 40 grams

Estimated GL 40x0.7*=28

This is high but if it was a meal out it would till be within your limit of 45, leaving 19 GL to spend as you wish.

* From the cheat sheet.

low GL diet for a while to compensate.

You could do it by introducing more high fibre, low glucose load foods from the lists.

In a nutshell: Maintenance means more carbs but you still need to control them. Do not go back to fat eating!

Increase your carbs slowly so you can remain in control

Chapter 8

Problem Solver

Estimating GLs for home cooking

You will have to estimate the GL of your baking from your ingredients by calculating the total GL for your batch and then the size of an allowed portion with a GL say of 5 or whatever GL you decide is appropriate.

This may seem like a lot of work but it only involves simple arithmetic and you will only have to do this once. Once you have the values for your normal baking, you will be able to add these to your chart.

First take the GL of 100 grams of each carbohydrate ingredient from my cheat sheet in appendix 1 and divide it by 100 to get the GL of one gram. Then multiply by the weight of that ingredient in the mix to get the total GL for the ingredient.

Next add all of these values together for all carbs to get the total GL for the bake.

In this example I have used odd numbers to illustrate the point but if you are dealing with a recipe which usually involves multiples or easy fractions of 100 then it is very easy to multiply or divide by the relevant fraction.

Ingredients	GL	
115 grams white flour	38	(115x33/100)
53 grams caster sugar	35	(53x66/100)
2 eggs	0	
Butter	0	
Total	73	

For large items like a cake or a tart, first calculate the number of GL 5 portions (assuming you are looking for GL5 portions) there are in the item as follows:-

Number of allowed portions N=Total GL for the item/5

In the example this is 73/5= 15 approximately. So divide your cake into 15 notional slices and one of these is for you. The rest can be divided in the normal way for others. In the future you will know how big a slice you are allowed.

If doing it by weight, which is more accurate, then calculate the allowed portion size as follows:-

Allowed portion size= Total weight of the item/N

Here I will use the approximate weight of the original ingredients in the example. You will use the weight of the finished cake.

Allowed portion size of the example recipe= 300/15 = 20 grams

If the product of the bake is a number of smaller items you can divide the average GL of each bun or tart, by 5 etc. to get the number of items you can eat, or what proportion of each item you can eat:-

Suppose we get 10 buns from our mix then the GL of each bun=73/10=7.3GL

Hence we can eat 5/7.3= 0.69 buns. Hardly worth the bother!

If you ate one whole bun you would be eating the equivalent of a 7.3 GL meal!

Further examples

In the examples below the calculations follow this format:- (total GL of items= (weight of items/ 100) x GL of 100 grams from the cheat sheet).

Traditional Latkes

5 large potatoes, ((160/100)x17)=1.6x17=27.2

1 large onion

3 egg

1/3 cup flour ((47/100)x33)=15.5

1 tsp. Salt

1/4 tsp. pepper

3/4 cup oil for frying Total GL=42.7

These are a high calorie food because of the combination of fat and carbohydrates and as we have already noted this is a deadly combination, However it is not the calories which concern us at the moment, but the glucose load. Assuming the recipe makes six latkes the GL of each latke is 42.7/6= 7.

Doughnuts -20 doughnuts

2 packages yeast

1/3 cup sugar ((67/100)x70)=47

3/4 cup water

1/4 cup orange juice =5

1/3 cup margarine

1/2 teaspoon salt

4 or 5 cups flour ((132/100)x33)=44

3 egg yolks

Jelly/jam of your choice for filling ((5/100)x70)=3.5

Powdered sugar for dusting the top = 0.5 approximately

The total GL here is: 47+5+44+3.5+0.5=100 GL

Average GL of one doughnut = (100/20)=5GL

Total GL of 5 doughnuts=25 GL

In a nutshell: Do some work on GL's of the food you normally use so that you can adjust the types and quantities in line with with your daily GL allowance before you start.

Managing carbs with normal family meals

If your family tend to have meals with a lot of carbs in them such as potatoes, pastry, sauces and commercial ice cream with perhaps tinned fruit in syrup. Managing this can be tricky.

You are going to have to make some choices and adjustments. In the main part of the meal, you may have to choose to forego the pastry and or the potato or both.

You can, of course, eat a GL 5 portion of potato and the contents of the pastry if this does not have any carb element, e.g. quiche tart. If you were eating out you may have some extra GL points to spend on a dessert.

As far as sauces and gravies go, you should score these as GL 5, per three hundred cc's or half a pint (4 servings), if they are thickened with flour, maize flour or potato starch. My researches suggest this is a good average, unless you make them essentially carb free by thickening with chick pea flour (gramm flour).

Ice cream is covered in the table in Appendix 1, unless you make your own and control the carb element. If the tinned fruit is in syrup, just pour off the syrup and wash the fruit in water before you take the fruit out and eat it. Remember unsweetened yoghurt is zero GL (150 grams) and it goes well with tinned fruit.

In a Nutshell: The way to handle family meals is to include as many options of low GL items as you can and max out on these. That way your family will not fret about you getting enough to eat.

Happy Holidays

If you are coming up to a series of celebrations, parties and holiday meals, take a run at this by reducing your GL limit for one or two days before the series of celebration days. If it is more than one day in a row do this for a several of days before. These are just sensible adjustments!

Obviously you will want to keep the carbs under control by maxing out on the low GL vegetables; protein and fat elements of the meals. In this way it is possible cope with celebration, and enjoy it, without putting on weight and even lose a pound or so. I doubt anyone will notice if you say 'Could I have some more turkey?' rather than 'Could I have some more potatoes?'

In a nutshell: Plan your approach to holidays and don't buy unnecessary high GL items in if you can help it. See Family meals above.

Too busy to cook

Typical question: I have an important high pressure job and, as a result, I eat a lot of convenience foods for speed. I don't have time to cook. What can I do?

Answer: It sounds as if you are taking work home. If your job requires you to do that, to the extent you can't cook a simple meal, you should consider a change of job.

Quite simply your job and eating habits are killing you. If the job is highly paid, use restaurants which will cater for your needs or get a cook. If it isn't highly paid enough to do that, what is in it for you?

Convenience foods contain large amounts of sugar as well as trans-fatty acids, which are deadly.

You can pre-cook many foods and keep them in the refridgerator to microwave later. Surely you could find some time on a weekend to cook some sausages, some salmon or tuna , or a couple of steaks! A large salad takes a few minutes to prepare, it will keep in the refridgerator for days, and is an anytime meal. This may not be a gourmet way of eating, but at least you have the assurance there is nothing nasty lurking in the food.

The last possibility is for you to move to an intermittent fasting regime. George Osborn, the former British Chancellor of the Exchequer, adopted this approach and visibly lost a lot of weight. See my book 'How To Start Intermittent Fasting A Simple Guide' (in press). Available soon on Kindle.

In a nutshell: To be too busy to do some simple cooking you should look at your life first and ask yourself if you really want to continue living like that. Try to cook wholesome food in advance or try intermittent fasting.

Skipping meals

Question: I am not a big breakfast eater and sometimes skip it. Wouldn't it accelerate my weight loss if I skip breakfast altogether?

Answer: Previously many authorities have advised against skipping breakfast, calling breakfast the most important meal of the day. This is partly because of what is known as the thermic effect of food (TEF), which is the boost to metabolic rates due to the energy needed to process food.

The theory was, by eating at least a small breakfast you raise you metabolic rate early, giving a metabolic advantage to the day. However, studies of the effect of a series of small meals against one or two meals show the same TEF.

Also your first meal of the day is, by definition, your breakfast. What does it matter it happens at 7 a.m. or 1 p.m.? Well 1 p.m. is better for weight control and is part of the scheme of intermittent fasting, for which see my book 'How To Start Intermittent Fasting A Simple Guide' (in press). Available soon on Kindle.

If you are not ready to eat when you first get up but tend to get hungry in mid morning, try to take your breakfast a short time later than usual or take a non-carb snack with you, such as some sausages or two hard boiled eggs.

In a nutshell: Skipping a meal can help reduce your insulin response and the easiest is breakfast. This can start you off into intermittent fasting.

Alcohol restrictions

Question: Why are there restrictions on alcohol use in the diet?

Let's begin with alcohol is a form of carbohydrate, it contains carbon, hydrogen and oxygen but its' metabolism is different.

Alcohol is a poison which has to be neutralised by the liver and in excess is bad for you! 92 to 98 percent of the alcohol absorbed by the digestive tract has to be dealt with by liver, which breaks it down eventually to more harmless chemicals.

As a first step, the liver breaks the alcohol down to acetaldehyde, which is even more toxic than alcohol and only then can it be made harmless. There are a lot of calories in alcohol, as many as seven per gram and when alcohol is broken down these have to be stored as fat.

Several studies have associated heavy alcohol consumption with the metabolic syndrome. Even light drinking (1 to 5 grams of alcohol a day) carries an increased risk of metabolic syndrome and the risk rises as the amount increases.

Moderate to large amounts of alcohol increase insulin resistance and increase the production of the bad cholesterol VLDL. That means if you imbibe large amounts of alcohol at meal times, more glucose will be circulating in the bloodstream, hence more insulin produced and, eventually, more glucose turned into fat. Small amounts e.g. a glass of red wine on the other hand are beneficial as I observed above.

In a nutshell: It is best to think of alcohol as pleasant but dangerous medicine, to be taken with extreme care.

Chapter 9

Other diets and the low GL diet

Low GL and low carb

Very low carbohydrate diets extend the fat burning time by as much as three to four times normal. This makes them an ideal starting point for initial weight loss. This makes a low carb program the first module which can be added to the diet.

If you are, having difficulty losing weight on this or any other diet you might be, 'insulin resistant' or quite simply unable to lose weight because of high resting levels of insulin, in which case a low carb/ high fat diet is the best starting point. See my book 'Starting a Low Carb Diet A Simple Guide'

As Westman, Phinney and Voleck, the authors of the 'New Atkins New You' point out, once weight loss has been achieved low GL carbs can be progressively introduced until weight starts to increase at which point you stop. In other words low carb morphs into low GL.

If you are not sure if you are insulin resistant then you see my companion book to this one 'Be Your own Diet Expert' available on Kindle.

Low GL and plant based diets

If you progressively lower the fat of content the low GL diet closer to the 10% recommended by the plant based diets while simultaneously increasing the leafy greens and pulses content, to keep the GL low, while replacing animal proteins with plant proteins you begin to move towards a plant based diet.

Introduce starch whole foods like rice, potatoes and grains and you will find yourself on a plant based diet.

A point in a meal would come, where you would find you were feeling full and well nourished with a sufficient calorie deficit to lose weight. That is where low GL morphs into plant based vegetarian diets.

Intermittent fasting

There are several versions of the intermittent fasting diet varying from fasting for three days occasionally through every other day to two days per week or just postponing breakfast and effectively eating only two meals a day.

The more days you fast the less you have to reduce your calorie intake on non fast days to produce the 10-20% deficit needed to lose weight safely.

All of these can be shown to produce a marked improvement in insulin resistance and blood markers for metabolic disease and so some form of intermittent fasting can be added to the diet either to augment it or as compensation for coming off the diet for a celebration. Just don't do too much.

In a nutshell: The low GL diet works well with other diets because it does not exclude all of their principles. It can morph into high fat/low carb or high carb/low fat and be used as a safe haven from both.

See my books 'Be Your Own Diet Expert', and 'How To Start Intermittent Fasting A Simple Guide' (in press). Available on Kindle.

Endtips

Tip: Eat a raw stick of celery before a meal. This will help to fill you and start your meal with valuable fibre.

Tip: Eat slowly, using a small fork or spoon helps this.

Tip: Avoid second helpings. Try to eat a satisfying amount with you first plateful.

Endwords

Whether we as individuals, who suffer from weight problems, face a fat or slim future is a matter of finding a whole life diet which promotes weight control and which we can stick with. It will never be a quick fix.

Then there are dietary supplements or diet pills. In recent years many natural products from cinnamon to exotic sounding chemicals such as conjugated linoleic acid and punicic acid have been linked to greater weight loss.

Consequently there has been a raft of companies who have jumped on the bandwagon to provide these types of supplement pills on line. Many of them are bogus and their pills contain little or none of the vital ingredient.

I have tried many of them and found no benefit. Their advertising often obscures scams whereby you think you are signing up for a free trial pack and you are actually signing up for an indefinite monthly supply at a very high price. Some of these pills contain actual poison and a woman in England died a few years ago from ingesting pills containing the poison dinitrophenol or DNP. My advice is to get started on an effective whole life diet now and forget about diet pills.

Scientists in the UK and US have started to identify 3 different types of individual, suited to different types of diet. The problem is they are not exactly the same three, although there is some overlap. Perhaps, in the future, an individual will be able to go to their doctor, answer a few questions, give a blood test and receive a personally tailored weight control program which suites their genetic makeup and lifestyle, but don't hold your breath.

When the mists clear on this we will have gone a long way in our quest to solve the obesity problem. In the meantime I commend this diet to you as the best way forward for a lot of people.

Thank you for downloading this book. I hope you have found it useful. If so will you please leave a review on Amazon which will help this book reach other readers.

Perhaps you would like to read one of my other books on various aspects of weight control, listed at the front of this book. I have tried to cover this topic in as easy to understand way as possible without undue reference to the science but rest assured all of this book rests on good science.

Good luck with your efforts. John

Contact John Rope: John.rope@sky.com

References

Note: In these references the word glycemic is science speak for glucose . I used Glucose load instead of glycemic load because that is what it refers to.

International Tables of Glycemic Index and Glycemic Load Values: 2008. Fiona S. Atkinson, RD, Kaye Foster-Powell, RD and Jennie C. Brand-Miller, PHD Diabetes Care 2008 Dec; 31(12): 2281-2283.

Dietary Fiber, Glycemic Load, and Risk of Non—insulin-dependent Diabetes Mellitus in Women Jorge Salmerón, MD; JoAnn E. Manson, MD; Meir J. Stampfer, MD; et al JAMA. 1997;277(6):472-477. doi:10.1001/jama.1997.03540300040031

Dietary glycemic load and colorectal cancer risk S Franceschi, LD Masco, L Augustin, E Negri… - Annals of Oncology, Volume 12, Issue 2, February 2001, Pages 173–178,

The effect of a low-carbohydrate, ketogenic diet versus a low-glycemic index diet on glycemic control in type 2 diabetes mellitus Westman, E.C., Yancy, W.S., Mavropoulos, J.C. et al. Nutr Metab (Lond) 5, 36 (2008) doi:10.1186/1743-7075-5-36

L. S. A. Augustin, S. Gallus, E. Negri, C. La Vecchia, Glycemic index, glycemic load and risk of gastric cancer, Annals of Oncology, Volume 15, Issue 4, April 2004, Pages 581–584,

Which Foods May Be Addictive? The Roles of Processing, Fat Content, and Glycemic Load Schulte EM, Avena NM, Gearhardt AN (2015). PLoS ONE 10(2): e0117959. https://doi.org/10.1371/journal.pone.0117959

Effect of a High-Protein, High-Monounsaturated Fat Weight Loss Diet on Glycemic Control and Lipid Levels in Type 2 Diabetes Barbara Parker, BSC, Manny Noakes, PHD, Natalie Luscombe, BSC and Peter Clifton, MD, PHD Diabetes Care 2002 Mar; 25(3): 425-430.

Dietary Glycemic Index, Glycemic Load, and Risk of Coronary Heart Disease, Stroke, and Stroke Mortality: A Systematic Review with Meta-AnalysisJingyao Fan, Yiqing Song, Yuyao Wang, Rutai Hui, Weili Zhang • journals plus.org December 20, 2012

Glycemic Index, Glycemic Load, and Thrombogenesis Jennie Brand-Miller1 , Scott Dickinson1 , Alan Barclay1 , Margaret Allman-Farinelli1 1Institute of Obesity, Nutrition and Exercise, and Department of Medicine, University of Sydney and Royal Prince Alfred Hospital, Camperdown, NSW, Australia

Semin Thromb Hemost 2009; 35(1): 111-118
ŵDOI: 10.1055/s-0029-1214154

A Low-Carbohydrate as Compared with a Low-Fat Diet in Severe Obesity Frederick F. Samaha, M.D., Nayyar Iqbal, M.D., Prakash Seshadri, M.D., Kathryn L. Chicano, C.R.N.P., Denise A. Daily, R.D., Joyce McGrory, C.R.N.P., Terrence Williams, B.S., Monica Williams, B.S., Edward J. Gracely, Ph.D., and Linda Stern, M.D. May 22, 2003 N Engl J Med 2003; 348:2074-2081 DOI: 10.1056/NEJMoa022637

Apendix 1

The GL Of Normal Foods

Foods with a normal portion GL of five or less

Please remember, until you have lost a significant amount of weight (30% of your target weight loss) avoid anything white, unless it is on this list.

Whichever foods you use, weigh out the allowed portion first time so that you know how big it should be. Take a photo or note a rule of thumb to remember it, e.g. 'about the size of an egg, or 'a small handful'.

Be careful not to mix up dry weight and wet weight with rice and cereal. Spray on fat, giving a thin film of fat for roasting is allowed.

If it isn't here it isn't allowed. Make your own list of your preferred and locally available food from these lists and use that to guide your shopping.

Take every opportunity to try low GL foods not on your list to expand your choice.

Remember zero rated vegetables are no limit so pile you plate to feel full and max out the fibre. Eat at least three portions a day.

I have included a summary of the foods which are permitted before you achieve your 30% weight reduction first. These are the foods you need to stock up on before you start depending on your preferences. The other lists can be consulted as required.

Summary: Zero to five glucose load foods you can eat right away

1.   All zero rated vegetables and fruits.

2.   All 5 GL vegetables and fruit not labelled as a special cases.

3.   Any meat.

4.   All cheeses, butter, cream etc.

5.   Any fish, prawns or other seafood.

6.Any Traditional Quorn (check for sugar in more recent products have added sugar.)

7. Tofu.

8. Cocoa can made with the milk allowances.

9. Herb teas- unlimited.

10.Milk whole fat or semi-skimmed- 500 ml.
11.Tomato juice pressed- no added sugar 250 ml.
12.Tea/coffee without sugar- unlimited, preferable

decaffeinated. 13.Soy/almond milk 1000 ml.
14.Water- unlimited!

15. Nuts and seeds from the list below.

Vegetables

All of these vegetables are zero rated on the diet

A. Artichoke, asparagus, aubergine.

B. Bamboo shoots- tinned, beetroot greens, broccoli, Brussels sprouts.

C. Cabbage-red, green and Savoy, carrots, cauliflower, celery, chard, collard greens, cress, courgette, cucumber.

D. Dandelion leaves.

F. Fennel.

K. Kale and all leafy green vegetables.

L. Lettuce.

M. Mushrooms-all types, mustard greens.

O. Okra, onions.

P. Palm hearts -tinned sliced, peppers sweet and hot, pumpkin.

R. Rocket leaves or other salad leaves.

S. Spring onions and shallots, squashes, spinach, Swiss chard.

T. Taro, tomato (in moderation) turnips mashed, turnip greens.

W. Water chestnuts.

Serve the salad greens with a tablespoonful of one of the following dressings: olive oil and vinegar or lemon, a French or Italian dressing- preferably Newman's Own, or balsamic vinegar. Also, try these dressings with hot food instead of a gravy or sauce!

Note: Peas, beans and other legumes are not included at first because the contain high amounts lectins. These are chemicals, rather like nerve agents, which are there to deter insect attack. Although they do not effect human beings in the same way they do interfere with the hormones of weight loss.

Acid fruits-

Have at lest five of these available all the time

Tick the ones you have now and put four or five of them on your shopping list every week.

A. Apricots raw

B. Blackberries, black currents blueberries, bilberries

C Cherries, cranberries, currents (fresh not dried),

G gooseberries, Grapefruit

K. Kiwi.

L Loganberries,

M. Melon.

O. Orange (not orange juice).

P. Plums just ripe peach- raw, pear raw.

R. Raspberries fresh.

S. Strawberries fresh.

W. Watermelon.

All of the above fruits are zero rated on the diet.

Foods which may be reduced to GL5

A * below means treat as 'special cases'.

Vegetables which can be GL5

Beetroot boiled, 80 grams, 3 ounces.

Corn/sweet corn boiled 40 grams- 1.5 ounces.*

Parsnips boiled or roasted with spray on fat 80 grams, 3 ounces.

Potato baked with skin 35 grams, 1.25 ounces.

Not to be eaten with fat (butter, cheese). *

Potato roasted with spray on fat 20 grams:*

Potato boiled 35 grams, 1.25 ounces.*!!

Swede boiled mashed- 140 grams 5 ounces.

Sweet potato boiled 40 grams. 1.5 ounces.*

Sweet potato- boiled or roasted with spray on fat 35 grams 1.25 ounces.*

Sweet potato- roasted in fat avoid.*

Note: Avoid fried or mashed potato or any other potato with added fat except as a special case.

If you any of eat these you must add GL 5 to your meal.. Portions are sometimes small! You may feel it is not worth eating them and replace them with low GL vegetables.

Bread

1/2 a burger bun.*

Pumpernickel average 25 grams, 1 ounce.*

White or wholemeal, whole grain, gluten free or specialist bread,15 grams (one slice), Again use as 'special cases'. *

Biscuits

Digestives 1 only. *

Crisp breads 11grams- 2 max. *

Oat cakes- 3 max.

Soda Rye crackers 10 grams 2 crackers. *

Cakes

Avoid.

Pastry

Avoid

Beverages/drinks

Cocoa can made with the milk allowances below.

Herb teas- unlimited.

Milk whole fat or semi-skimmed- 500 ml.

Tomato juice pressed- no added sugar 250 ml.

Unsweetened, cranberry juice 250 ml *

Tea/coffee without sugar- unlimited, preferable decaffeinated.

Soy/almond milk 1000 ml.

Water- unlimited!

Dairy/Soya products

Ice cream- no sugar 20 grams, 3/4 ounce.*

Ice cream- premium, made from cream and full fat milk 50 grams, 1.5 ounces.

Almond milk 1000 ml.

Soya yoghurt 250ml.

Milk whole fat or semi-skimmed- 500 ml.

Bananas just ripe 1/2.

Fruit fresh

Alll acid Frits listed above.

Serving size 35-50 grams. Eat two portions a day

Other fruit -

Add 5 to daily total GL each time

Apples 120 grams, 4 ounces.

Grapes 120 grams, 4 ounces. *

Mango raw 120 grams, 4 ounces. *

Peaches raw 120 grams, 4 ounces. *

Peaches canned in light syrup.- 120 grams, 4 ounces. Pour off the syrup and rinse in water.*

Pears raw 120 grams, 4 ounces.

Pears in juice or syrup- 120grams, 4 ounces. Pour off the syrup and rinse in water*

Prunes 5 grams, 0.15 ounces. Pour off the syrup and rinse in water*

Cereals

GL 5- not to be eaten until you have lost 30% of your target weight.

Oats (porridge) 30 grams, 1 ounce dry weight. *

Albran 15 grams, 0.5 ounces dry weight. *

Muesli (no sugar) or home made with oats, nuts and seeds-15 grams, 0.5 ounces dry weight. *

Bran buds 20 grams, 0.6 ounces dry weight. *

Grains

GL 5- not to be eaten until you have lost 30% of your target weight.

Pearled Barley 60 grams, 2 ounces dry weight.

Quinoa 60 grams, 2 ounces dry weight. *

Bulgar 60 grams, 2 ounces dry weight. *

Semolina 60 grams, 2 ounce wet weight. *

Rice white, brown, wild- 30 grams, 1 ounce dry weight. *

Rice Brown 30 grams, 1 ounce dry weight. *
Rice wild 3 grams, 1 ounce dry weight. *

Rice,, wild- 30 grams, 1 ounce dry weight. *

Nuts and seeds-

Use for snacks and add to salads and muesli. Add GL 3 to your total each time.

Almonds, whole and ground- 20 whole nuts, 2 tablespoons ground.

Brazils - 3 nuts.

Cashews- 4 nuts- not in the first 2-3 weeks.

Coconut, shredded unsweetened- 1/2 cup.

Macademia- 4 nuts.

Hazelnuts- 20 nuts.

Peanuts- 30 nuts.

Pecans- 8 nuts.

Pistachios- 20 nuts.

Various seeds- pumpkin, sesame, sunflower etc. 2 tablespoons.

Various butters made from these nuts and seeds, 1 tablespoon= GL 2.5 (except cashew butter which is best avoided 1 tablespoon=GL5).

Cheat Sheet

The following are averages for the four common carb ingredients of home and restaurant food and some of their most common derivatives rounded down for safety. Use this only when you have lost 30% of your desired weight.

Ingredient	GL per 100 grams	GL5 Portion g
Bread bun/bagel	30	16
Bread sliced	33	14
Brd slice no gluten	33	14
Flour (all)	33	NA
Sugars (all)	70	NA
Potato (all methods)*	26	17
Rice all types*	26	17
Pasta (all types)*	31	15
French Fries/chips**	17	16**
Noodles (All types)	31	15
Pizza (all types)	19	14**
Pastry (all types)**	27	12**

*Cooked weight

**Reduced because of fat/carb combo

In order to make use of this sheet you will need to be thoroughly familiar with the size of one hundred grams for the relevant food type and with the size of a GL 5 portion.

Therefore if you want to eat any form of potato then 26 grams is your maximum safe portion size, whether the potatoes are boiled or baked. Get to know what this looks like and you can eat potatoes safely anywhere. If in doubt cut the portion in half!

Similarly if you know the total weight of an ingredient then you can get a quick estimate of the GL of that ingredient by its weight, relative to its one hundred grams GL above. So if you have two hundred and fifty grams of flour, you have an estimated GL of 2.5x33=83 approximately. See " Estimating GLs for home cooking" below.

In a nutshell: Start by scoring your most common meals for GL and make necessary adjustments to reduce their GL. You will soon be able to look at a meal and estimate how much of each of the constituent foods you can eat. Increasing some and reducing others can give a fulfilling meal which is also slimming.

Appendix 2

Some sample low GL meals

These can be added to as you experiment with low GL foods and find other favourites. They can be mixed and matched and you can of course go beyond the limits of the diet if circumstances or common sense dictate. I do not expect you to stick to these guidelines as if they were written on tablets of stone. My aim to make your aware of the impact of certain foods on your body and to become a good assessor of which foods are the better choice, especially in circumstances where the choice is limited as in a restaurant.

Breakfast

Two boiled or fried eggs

Omelette or scrambled egg with or without your choice of, mushrooms, onions or any of the zero rated vegetables.

Two Qourn chicken fillets or original sausage.

Smoked salmon. Delicious in scrambled egg.

A cheese salad.

Water if you are planning to delay breakfast or skip it.

Lunch Light Snack

Two Quorn chicken slices or chicken breasts wrapped in a lettuce leaf.

Two Quorn or whole meat sausages wrapped in a lettuce leaf.

A piece of cheese.

A small salad.

Dinner/ Lunch Main meal

Any meat (no more than 6 ounces-170 grams, not in a sauce and cooked from raw) with low GL vegetables like cabbage, broccoli, cauliflower or any of the low GL vegetables.

Low carb sausage, egg and bacon.

Salad with cold meat, Quorn slices, eggs or cheese.

Omelette.

Water if you are planning to skip lunch.

Tea/ Supper

A small portion of ketogenic bread or cake made with almond or coconut flour. There are many recipes on the internet. I have put two of my favourites after this appendix.

Strawberries (or any other berries) and cream.

Small portion of yoghurt.

A light version of breakfast.

Add Xyitol or similar sweetener to taste but try to keep the sweetness as low as possible until you have phased out sweetness from your life. See my companion volume 'Sugar Free-Dom: How To Kick The Sugar Demon Out Of Your Life.' Available on Kindle and Amazon.

Sweet or pudding course

Strawberries, yoghurt etc as above.

Chia seed puddings.

Chia seeds are tiny little seeds which absorb water avidly to form a jelly like substance with the seeds suspended in it like semolina but with no carbs. Thes can be sweetened with a sweetener if you must. Soak them overnight in whole milk, or almond to coconut milk to make a delicious sweet for the next day. If you suffer from constipation a chia seed sweet is the gentle answer. Only one per day is recommended.

Any 5 GL fruit portion or, if it is the end of your eating day, you can go wild and have more than the normal permitted amount.

Snacks

Half portion of any of the above breakfast or light lunch suggestions.

Two hard boiled eggs

Very Low Carb Bread

From a recipe on the Ketoconnect website.

Very low carb or keto bread tends to be dense and this bread achieves its fluffiness from separating the eggs into yolks and whites and whipping the whites until they form fluffy peaks. This give the bread a lighter more bread like texture and makes it taste more bread like.

Prep timer 10 minutes

Cooking Time 30 minutes

Total Time   40 minutes

Servings 20. Calories per serving 90 cal

Ingredients

1 1/2 cups almond flour (finely ground).

6 large eggs separated.

!/4 cup butter melted.

3 tsp baking powder.

1/4 tsp cream of tartar -can leave out.

1 pinch sea salt.

6 drops liquid stevia -optional

Method

- Preheat oven to 375.

- Separate the egg whites from the yolks. Add Cream of Tartar to the whites and beat until soft peaks are achieved.

- In a food processor combine the egg yolks, 1/3 of the beaten egg whites, melted butter, almond flour, baking powder and salt (Adding ~6 drops of liquid stevia to the batter can help reduce the mild eggy taste). Mix until combined. This will be a lumpy thick dough until the whites are added.

- Add the remaining 2/3 of the egg whites and gently process until fully incorporated. Be careful not to over-mix as this is what gives the bread it's volume!

- Pour mixture into a buttered 8x4 loaf pan. Bake for 30 minutes. Check with a toothpick to ensure the bread is cooked through. Enjoy! 1 loaf makes 20 slices.

I recommend this website for all kinds of low carb food with easy to prepare recipes. Go to the website https://www.ketoconnect.net for more information.

Very Low Carb Vanilla Cake

This comes from the website 'Sweet as honey'

Note this is for one layer.

Prep time 25 minutes. Cook time 30 minutes.

No of slices 12.

Ingredients

Vanilla cake

2 cups almond flour 240 g (finely ground).

4. eggs

1/2 cup sugar free crystal sweetener. Erythritol or xylitol.

2 tablespoonfuls coconut oil (melted and allowed to cool slightly) or avocado or almond oils.

1 teaspoon baking powder

1 tsp vanilla extract

Vanilla butter cream frosting

1/2 cup 150g dairy free butter or unsalted butter. Out of the fridge for four hours

3 cups powdered sweetener erythritol or xylitol

1 tsp vanilla

3 tablespoons coconut cream or heavy cream

Method

- Preheat oven to 160C (325F). Grease a 9 inches round cake pan with coconut oil or butter. Set aside.

- In a large mixing bowl, whisk eggs with sugar free sweetener, oil and vanilla. Process as if you whisk a breakfast omelette. It should not take more than 30 seconds-1 minute, all you want is to combine the ingredients together.

- Whisk in almond flour and baking powder and whisk until evenly combined.

- Pour the vanilla cake batter into the prepared pan.

- Bake for 25 minutes, in the center of your oven, fan-bake mode is ideal if you have one otherwise use regular mode. Your cake is cooked when a skewer inserted in the middle of the cake come out clean or with few to no crumbs on it.

- Cool 5 minutes in the pan then release the cake on a cooling rack. Cool for 1 or 2 hours before adding the frosting or enjoy plain.

Layer vanilla cake

- Repeat the vanilla cake recipe one more time to create a second vanilla cake

- Make sure you clean, dry and grease again the cake pan before baking the second cake.

Buttercream frosting

- Add the soft butter cubes and vanilla in a stand mixer. Make sure you use the paddle attachment. Mix on high speed until it forms a pale, smooth and fluffy butter.

- Reduce to low speed and gradually add the sugar free powdered sweetener, half a cup at a time. When all the sugar free sweetener has been added, mix on medium speed for 2 minutes until it forms a fluffy cream.

- Add cream and keep whisking for 1 minute to incorporate.

- Spread the frosting between the 2 cake layers and on sides using a icing spatula. Watch the video on the website to learn how to frost your layer cake easily.

- Place the cake in the fridge for 2 hours to set up the frosting if desired.

- Note: If only frosting one half of the cake halve the frosting ingredients.
Go to the website.- https://www.sweetashoney.co

How To Steam Eggs

Eggs are a most important low carb food. All the scare mongering which went on in the 1980s and 1990s was just hot air. Eating up your four or five eggs a day is not going to put your cholesterol up! If you take some in your body makes less. So eat more eggs and keep your carbs down!

This method gives you between two and twenty hard boiled eggs to keep in the fridge and use for meals or snacks ad lib.

If you don't do any cooking the method is very simple but it means you must keep an eye on things for 8 minutes and I am sure you can do that.

First decide how many eggs you want to cook and find a pan which looks big enough to take them. It must have a lid.

Place about 1/4 inch of water in the pan and put on the heat with the lid on.

When the water boils place the eggs gently in the pan, replace the lid, put back on the heat and bring to the boil.

Time for eight minutes, remove form the heat and fill the pan with cold water to stop further cooking. Cooking is that easy.

Acknowledgements

My thanks to my wife Barbara who has proof read and edited the book with great skill.